Life After Work

Retirement Books

Susan Kersley

Published by Susan Kersley, 2024.

LIFE AFTER WORK

©Susan Kersley

First edition 2021

Updated 2024

While we have taken every precaution in preparing this book, the publisher assumes no responsibility for errors or omissions, or for damages resulting from the use of the information contained.

Table of Contents

Copyright Page 1

1. Life transition 6

2. New Routines 12

3. Rethink your life 18

4. Will you be bored? 24

5. Communicate effectively 26

6. Life after work 31

7. Plans into action 34

8. Ways to stay busy 38

9. Finding your purpose 40

10. Get sorted 43

11. Myths about retirement 49

12. Opportunities in life after work 54

13. Make life easier 58

14. The advantages of retiring 61

15. Personal experience 67

Finally 68

"What lies behind us, and what lies before us are tiny matters compared to what lies within us." – Ralph Waldo Emerson

1. Life transition.

Retirement is a time to decide how to spend the rest of your life. It isn't the end of the road. It's your life after work.

It's time to reassess your life and decide how to spend the rest of it. You may find, when you retire, that you feel exhausted and it's difficult to motivate yourself to do anything except sit around, eat and watch television.

Although it's fine to relax when you retire, you rem**ain fitter and healthier** if you **develop new interests, make new friends and go to places you have never been to before.**

Ending your working life is an important transition. It means giving up the identity that has become an ingrained part of who you are. It's possible that your persona dominated.

Whatever the reason for your retirement, whether it was a planned decision or forced on you because of redundancy, ill health or dismissal, it's usual to have a reaction to the change in your status.

You may be happy about leaving a job you didn't enjoy. You may grieve when you move from being employed to retired.

Changing your identity is a fresh experience and with this comes sadness, guilt, anger and eventually acceptance and moving on. It's part of the process.

Retirement is a chance to change your life. This can energise you unless you dread the changes that occur when your work routine no longer dominates your life. You have opportunities opening if you recognise them. It's up to you: if you do nothing, then nothing changes. If you follow where your heart leads, your world can be your oyster.

You may plan to do many things when you retire, but unless you have savings or a decent pension, you may not afford to do all you would like unless you earn some extra money.

Retirement is a chance to start anew. If your job involved being very logical, then something more creative may excite you. Perhaps you've always enjoyed making things, taking photographs, drawing and painting, or making music. Is this the beginning of a new career? It all depends what you want.

Talk to retired people. Notice who seems to be happy and enjoying life, and who talks about missing work. You can learn from the first group and make your own decision.

When **choosing a career after retirement**, do what you love. It's fine to relax when you retire. However, you remain fitter and healthier if you **develop new interests,** make new friends and visit places you have never been to before.

Will you **explore new opportunities**? You may have abilities you weren't aware of before. Be brave and find them!

Retirement is a time for change. Do you prefer to spend your time alone or with others? Would you like to get paid or volunteer to help people in your community? Would you like to be fitter? Do you like working out?

List what you wished you had time for when you were working.

- What stops you from doing those things now?
- Are you in the right place?
- Do you have the correct skills?

Your **self-esteem may be low** if you believe you can only do things related to your work experience. However, when you retire you can develop the confidence and courage to try something new. It might surprise you to find you have hidden talents and abilities. Doing something different is energising and opens your mind to many possibilities.

Will you explore fresh places or satisfy long held dreams?

- Reassess your life.
- Decide what you want.
- Take the first steps.

If you have worked in the same profession since university, or school, break away from your familiar mould.

Maturity comes to us all with age. But retirement isn't the end of the road. Not at all. You may be aware soon after you finish your working life that there is an air of excitement about many people when they talk of all they plan to do during their retirement years. You may approach this phase of life with a mixture of expectation and apprehension, coping with life with less routine and the opportunities it brings to put your ideas into practice.

It's time to come to terms with not having to achieve everything. It's about your own ageing and eventual mortality. Recognise what you can and can't do. However, it's not a time to sit back and fall into a heap in the corner. Nor is it time to raise your hands and drop your head in a resigned way and do absolutely nothing. It's the time to recognise changes that happen, whatever your age, when you stop working. If you are apprehensive about what the future has in store, seeing the funny side of life is important.

There is life after work, and you can decide what sort of life it will be.

Transformation can seem scary. You decide if you will make any changes. Life is like a spreadsheet. Change one thing, and everything else changes! When you **change your daily pattern** of activities, you become different in other people's eyes; they behave differently towards you.

Is change always better? That's an interesting question to consider. Things will change for the better, when you stop doing what you don't like and do more of what you love to do. It's about **attitude of mind** and deciding that things will improve and then making those things happen.

Years ago, retirement was the end of the road. You would have a party: your work colleagues gave you a clock and good wishes and they sent you off to laze about and do nothing. There would be jokes about wishing they could spend all day in a bed or in front of the telly and that would be it. You would probably have done exactly that, eaten too much, maybe drunk too much, exercised too little and eventually come to an untimely end. Not a happy picture, was it?

Things are different these days. Maybe you retired before the statutory retirement age. Maybe they made you redundant.

Did a health issue force you to take early retirement? Have you left your job to satisfy a lifelong yearning to do something entirely different?

It's challenging and sometimes scary to enter any new phase of life, and dealing with transition and change can have challenges. When you prepare for retirement and the change it brings, it helps if you plan for the emotional roller coaster you may experience.

Retirement is not the end, but the beginning of new opportunities.

You can enjoy life so much more if you have a **positive mental outlook.** When things don't happen the way you want, look at what you learned so you don't make the same mistakes. If the same situation happens again, you can react more effectively. **Be a glass half full** rather than a glass half empty person. If something doesn't work out the way you hoped, decide what you would do differently.

If you had to leave work unplanned because of ill health, or suspension for malpractice, then you may be upset and confused about what's happening. You may be angry about how life treated you, or guilty about something you did, which became much bigger than you imagined it could.

It is possible to appreciate life again amidst the negative aspects. It's important to **enjoy life** and see the funny side of situations that upset you. Step back and find an individual or a group to support you during the tough times. Others who have been through similar situations give you words of comfort and guidance. It's reassuring to realise that others have been through similar experiences.

If you become bothered about something or someone, try picturing the person as a cartoon character or a clown. Imagine them speaking with a squeaky voice or singing everything. It may surprise you how doing this can diminish the anger or frustration you were feeling about what happened.

Make a joke of it, by telling the story to someone else, or picturing it in your mind's eye, you change your perception.

2. New Routines.

If you are someone who enjoyed the security of regular work, then you may find the prospect of retirement and losing that reassurance and routine somewhat daunting and be feeling a loss of confidence about how you'll cope without those patterns to your days.

Develop a new routine and make changes to enjoy the freedom of retirement.

Regain your self-confidence as you plan your days. Retirement is an opportunity to do many things you didn't have time or inclination to do while you were working.

Set goals. When you have something to work towards, your confidence increases. This may be to complete a project at home. Set a time frame to work on it or an amount to do each day in order to experience the task completed. Working to a deadline, even if this is self-imposed, rather than boss imposed, enables you to fulfil your tasks.

Discover extra activities. Don't sit around hoping something will arrive in your lap. Instead, be open to fresh experiences and new things.

Retirement is a time to enjoy hobbies. You might have wanted to learn a language, or sing or play a musical instrument. As you do new things with a positive intention of learning, your confidence increases and your outlook and enjoyment of life soars.

Excitement is the way you feel that first week or two of not working. Elation about leaving 'that place' and never having to be answerable to 'those people' any more. As you remember some of 'those things' that were the last straw which resulted in you deciding to stop, resign or take early retirement, you may feel quite angry about the way people behaved towards you over the years. You gave your all yet had very little recognition for what you did. Now you have the last laugh, don't you? They will have to manage without you, with a replacement who won't know the job.

A sense of laziness may set in when you mooch around the house all day, not really wanting to do anything much, perhaps regretting that you left. However, because you are retired, others believe you are at their beck and call. It's important you are aware of this possibility and you do what you want for others, but not so much that you no longer have the time to follow your own interests and hobbies.

Nevertheless, starting every day with absolutely no idea what you plan to do is not likely to result in achieving your dreams or your purpose. You can have wonderful dreams of what you would like, but when you plan specifically then you find that time passes more quickly than you could imagine. You have all the time in the world when you retire. But is this true? No, you have the time you have. Full stop. You don't know what the future may bring you. You don't know how long it may be before you cannot do the things you want to do.

Without the schedules of work, you have the chance to make more choices, especially in the way you want to use each day.

This may include more involvement with friends and family. You may decide to look after your grandchildren or become involved as a volunteer helping at a local playgroup. If you haven't any grandchildren of your own, you could offer to become a substitute grandparent to children who have none.

Consider how you want to spend your days when you are retired. You no longer have to go to work each day, so be careful of filling your day with other obligations that you don't want. You may be a person who only wants to do things for other people and is happy to be of use to them. That is absolutely fine so long as you are not avoiding the possibility of doing new and exciting things, too.

When people ask you to do something, consider if you really want to say 'yes' or 'no'. If you decide to help, then be clear with that person whether they believe you are promising to doing this every day, each week or regularly. If so, do you want to have that commitment?

It might be a relief to have something to do regularly. You might resent your agreement if new opportunities come your way. Being retired is a lot about finding a balance between your responsibilities to others and obligations to yourself. That's why it's important to spend some time sorting these in your own mind to clarify how to respond to others who want to use your time and energy and which might result you having less of both to use for your personal retirement projects.

It's not a matter of all or nothing. There is a middle way when you can do things for others and spend part of your day in doing those things but also having plenty of time, energy and motivation for yourself.

Have you ever tried wearing a different sort of shoe in order to be like others? Once I wore flip-flops during a holiday and my feet objected strongly until they got used to the unfamiliar sensation. My feet were unaccustomed to the extra pressures of the flip-flop's straps because they were more used to being enclosed in socks and town shoes, and they reacted to the flip-flops with several blisters. However, I knew that after a few days, the skin would heal and the skin adapt to their new footwear.

Life in retirement can be like adapting to flip-flops. At first, doing something different may feel strange and tempt you to stop and abandon whatever it is which caused the discomfort. However, when you persist, the scars heal and you adapt to the new situation.

As you prepare to retire or adapt to the transition called retirement, there will be many opportunities to do something different. Be brave and go ahead. Take the opportunities which retirement brings even if it seems as though you won't be able to accept your new lifestyle and miss the routines of work too much. It's not just the schedule you miss at first, it may be the camaraderie of the workplace and the friendships connected with working together.

When you retire, you need **to fill the gap** caused by losing these things. Although you may keep in contact with workplace friends, the friendships, were, to a large extent, related to common work experiences.

When you **develop new habits** in retirement, you find you meet new people and **develop other interests.** At first, you must make these changes consciously because they may seem strange as you plan your day in exciting ways.

Most things need repeating at least twenty-one times to become automatic. Be aware of what you want to achieve in your retirement and move your sights forward to the new opportunities retirement offers you.

If you miss the work routine, you can either find another job, or sign on for a course and learn whatever you missed out on earlier in your life. Just remember to keep your goal in mind and don't give up too soon.

If the thought of losing your working-day routine worries you and you wonder how you will pass your days without it, then take heart. There are new opportunities that open up for you depending on what you really would like to do during your retirement. Some people are very anxious about their loss of income and want to find some other suitable employment, which could be entirely different from their previous occupation.

Whatever you decide to do, avoid putting yourself into a stressful situation. It's very important to enjoy yourself and find plenty to do each day. A common experience of retired people is that they discover things they didn't know were available to them and their days fill up, so much and they say: 'I'm so busy now, I don't know how I ever had time to work!'

As always, **it is about balance** between what you do for yourself and what you do because of pressure from others. If you can equalise your time and energy, the better for you. Be aware of your internal reactions to doing things you love against doing something because of an obligation. If the latter leaves you feeling drained or stressed, then it is very important to confront this and make adjustments so that what you do gives you a feeling of excitement and anticipation.

What have you neglected while working? Now is the time to address those parts of your life.

When you **discover the joys of retirement** and the wonderful opportunities, it offers to experience a long and healthy retirement for many years.

3. Rethink your life.

Retirement is an opportunity to re-think your life and do something different. You can find new things to do that you've been putting off for years and know that it's the time to make up for lost opportunities and get on with what you want to do.

Get fit, because as you become older, you may be prone to illnesses and you may deteriorate physically and mentally too. To delay the changes as long as you can, it's important to look after yourself and make up for years of lack of self-care when you were working.

Exercise every day, because keeping your body moving and your muscles and joints in excellent condition are vital for remaining fit and well as long as you can. It also helps recovery if you become ill.

The best sort of exercise as you get older is **walking.** If you take a walk most days for about half an hour, you will keep your heart beating efficiently. Besides walking, yoga helps you to relax, and enables your joints and muscles to function well. They say that yoga affects your mind too, and that a flexible body relates to a flexible mind.

Keep your mind active: You can read all the books you never had the time for in the past. You can join a class to get up to date with computers and the internet, or a club that meets socially and has regular informative talks.

Keep your mind active because challenges are present each day. Retirement, like the rest of life, is an ongoing learning experience. Don't expect to know all the answers right away. When you know the question, you will search for the answer. Plan what you want. You may need to go to a specialist such as a financial advisor or a solicitor.

You know what you want already. This knowing may hide in your subconscious mind, your inner self. You discover new things about yourself and your purpose as you go through this transition.

Have fun. Enjoy this part of your life. See the fun side of life and laugh frequently.,

Concentrate on eating plenty of fresh fruit and vegetables and avoid ultra-processed food. Keep a balance between the different food groups. These are: protein such as meat, fish, eggs, beans, nuts, pulses and seeds and soya products such as tofu; complex carbohydrates such as whole grains, wheat, barley, oats, corn, rice; and healthy oils such as olive oil and coconut oil, in moderation.

Eat healthy meals because you feel better and lower your risk of illness. You have more energy and can enjoy life. It's easy to get into a habit of over-eating once you retire.

Part **of keeping fit** during retirement is eating sensibly while also indulging from time to time in a little of what you fancy. Strict diets are definitely out, but eating plenty of fruit and vegetables, low fat protein and complex carbohydrate and the healthier fat from olives, avocado and nuts, can only do you good and help to prevent illness.

Eat plenty of healthy foods in order to avoid falling into the trap of living on bread and jam. If you don't enjoy cooking, there are places that offer activities and a hot meal, and pubs that have inexpensive meals for pensioners. However, it's easy to eat simple things which are healthy and cheap, for example baked beans on toast or baked potato and grated cheese with salad are healthy and will fill you up and are better for you than junk food.

Cut out any poisons that you can control, such as smoking, excessive alcohol or food additives. Only take prescribed medication and understand your options and potential side effects. Basic health advice is to stop smoking or expect to develop a smoking related illness during the early years of your retirement.

Retirement can feel like a long holiday, and on holiday you may drink more. However, you are not on holiday and it's best for your general health to keep your alcohol intake below the recommended levels for health.

Keep your body well exercised when you retire. Whatever your age or physical ability, you will benefit from exercise. It doesn't have to be high powered. In fact, the best forms of exercise, whatever your age, are walking, swimming, dancing, yoga, pilates or a combination of these. The most important things are that it is regular and you enjoy yourself.

Plan when, where, and what. The trouble is that when you retire, you may either take on too many activities or not find the time to exercise or do nothing and sit around feeling sorry for yourself. Resolve to do some exercise for at least half an hour on most days.

Even though you may do less than you could years ago, it is vital to keep moving and stretching to keep healthy. Yoga and walking are good for these outcomes.

Exercise every day and make sure you walk, do an exercise class, go to the gym, or swim. It doesn't matter what you decide to do for so long you enjoy and can do easily, so you keep your heart healthy and your body fit and flexible. Exercise must be an important part of your new daily or weekly routine. It doesn't have to be 'over the top.' It just needs to be something you can fit into your lifestyle. Choose an exercise you enjoy without due stress.

Walking is one of the easiest ways to achieve this. You can do it every day by going out of your front door, with no special equipment. Do it anywhere, on your own or with company. Do more walking when before you would have driven your car, or if you go by bus walk to the next bus-stop.

Always take the stairs instead of a lift and don't begrudge any walking that is necessary during your day. Do this in the countryside, beside the sea or in a park. These might add benefits of getting away from polluted air in towns and cities. Walking, yoga and swimming are ways to help your health and well-being for a life after work.

Exercise is vital to do regularly because while not actually preventing any illness it will keep you well for longer, with your heart beating strongly, your joints more mobile and your body more flexible and able to cope with whatever happens as you get older and so if you become ill your chance of a speedy recovery increases.

Keep your joints and muscles active with regular walking, and stretching and exercise, which increase your heart rate such as swimming, dancing, exercising to music or tennis.

If you want to be with others, then have a walk with someone or find out about local classes, whether these are for exercise at your local gym or for class activities such as dancing or yoga.

Going to the Gym: a good way to tone your muscles and get fitter if you can put up with the cost and monotony of exercising on machines!

Swimming: Your swimming pool or the sea is waiting for you to swim your lengths and is an ideal form of non-weight bearing exercise. Go for it.

Dancing: What do you fancy? Learning new dances? Or going back to your youth with rock and roll, jive and samba? Keep active and enjoy how invigorated you feel when you move to a great beat on the radio or go out for the evening with friends.

Yoga is the greatest way to stretch all parts of your body, keep moving and getting the benefit of exercise and relaxation at the same time. It's been around for hundreds of years and you can benefit too. Pilates is good for this too.

Golf: If you love golf, then retirement brings you the chance to indulge your sport of choice. If you don't like golf, then you don't have to have a white ball in order to walk a distance. There are places apart from golf courses for walking.

Drive less: Keep your physical fitness as good as you can by regular exercise, and this includes using your car less. You have the advantage of senior rail cards and bus passes, if you live in the UK, so use these and enjoy visiting fresh places instead of driving. Using public transport more often also encourages you to walk more and thus benefits your health too.

After you have exercised, also relax. This can be done sitting in a chair or lying down for a few minutes. Think about each part of your body and tense and then relax it from your feet to your head and as you do this think about letting go of tension and allowing the muscles to relax. Then let everything be completely relaxed for a few moments as you breathe in and out slowly and allow your body to recover from the exercise.

4. Will you be bored?

Do what you enjoy. This is most important because retirement is a time for you to have fun and stop doing things which frustrate, annoy or upset you. When you were working, you probably had to do things you didn't want to do, but in retirement you have choices. If there is something that has to be done and you don't want to do it, get someone else to do it. Pay someone for gardening or housework or swop with a friend so you help each other.

Retirement is a time to finish projects you started years ago, to get your clutter sorted and to do things you didn't get around to before.

There may be **activities** you wished you'd done previously. These might include travel to countries you've not visited before, learning a foreign language or a musical instrument. Take an Open University course There are plenty of courses available, or find what you are looking for at your local adult education centre.

Lifelong learning is extremely important, so keep your mind and body as active as possible.

Take up neglected hobbies you've enjoyed in the past. Retirement gives you the chance to revisit these.

There may be **skills** you have but you didn't have the time for. You can revisit your chosen hobby or interest.

LIFE AFTER WORK 25

Join in with your local community. Get involved and contribute because you are at a stage in your life when you have a lot to offer and can help others.

Meet old **friends** regularly and make new ones too, so you don't stay at home feeling sorry for yourself. If you have friends who are also retired, meet regularly. Meeting people for a walk, a cup of tea or sharing a meal together helps to keep boredom away.

Keep in touch with **family,** whether they live nearby or on the other side of the world. They may be busy but don't let that stop you picking up the phone, sending emails or talking on-line.

5. Communicate effectively.

To effectively communicate, we realise we are all different in the way we perceive the world and use this understanding as a guide to our communication with others. Anthony Robbins

Communication is listening and speaking. Listen and understand what someone is saying. Be clear about what you are asking or telling them.

It's important to **communicate effectively.** If you are about to make dramatic changes in your life, explain why you are about to behave differently. Even though they will expect you to change, they also presume you to be the same. If you plan to stop doing things you've been doing for ages or start doing something you haven't done before, tell others because they will notice differences in you.

Too many people don't talk about what they want to do because they assume others would not approve. By communicating your intentions, you will help to prepare others for what you intend to do.

As you adapt to your change of routine, others get accustomed to the transformations in you. They may not understand so it's important to talk to those affected.

Too many people don't get as far as talking about what they would like to do because they assume that some people would be upset or not approve of what they want to do. By communicating your intentions, you will help to prepare others for your changed way of life when you retire.

First and most important is to **get into rapport**. If you think they may not like what you are going to say, start with something positive, then tell them something negative, and finish with something positive.

If people don't seem to hear or understand what you say, learn to **listen twice as much as you speak**. (Two ears and one mouth!). Understand their point of view because they are more likely to give you the attention and consideration you want. When you show understanding to them, then they are more likely to give you the attention and consideration you want.

'Mirroring and matching' are skills that help you communicate effectively. You do this when you get along well with someone. Mirror the other person's body posture. Although this may seem more difficult at first, you discover that when you copy the same posture and movements, there will be a greater level of rapport. The important thing is to do this subtly. Match their breathing rate and their tone of voice, too.

Notice the type of language they use. Is it visual, auditory, or kinaesthetic? Use the same language in reply. If they use mainly visual words, reply using the same. Ask 'Do you see what I mean?' Auditory people use words such as 'I hear what you say.' Kinaesthetic people use emotional language such as 'I feel it and I know what I have to do.'

Be interested in the other person, to understand their world and their point of view. Imagine what it might be like if you could 'get into their shoes' and see how you might look from their eyes.

Use your body to communicate by adopting a strong, relaxed, open posture, centred and ready for action, as in martial arts. Stand with your knees slightly apart and bent.

Make sure your **body language is open** because your body speaks its own language. Sitting with your arms folded and legs crossed gives out a negative message compared with an open body posture.

Poor communication may be simply because you don't speak clearly or are using complicated words, nor saying precisely what it is you want to convey.

People like compliments more than insults and are likely to respond to you when they feel you appreciate them. End with a positive statement, even if the rest of the exchange between you was negative, because the other person will remember how the end of the conversation.

People often misunderstand each other, especially if they are not fully listening to what is being said and jump to conclusions too easily. **Make sure they understand** what you are asking them to do because they may not have heard you properly. They may have heard the start of what you were saying and then had their own assumptions about what you were asking them.

At the end of the conversation, **sum up your discussion** because it's easy to remember the end of a discussion and forget the beginning. Summarise by saying this is what we discussed, and this is what will happen now.

Develop confidence and self-belief by stating clearly your request, or what you would like the other person to do without excuses or reasons, because some people get inundated in explanation.

Don't say 'you make me cross'. Instead, acknowledge your emotions by saying 'when you do that, I feel cross,' so you take back ownership of your reactions and take personal responsibility for them.

Listen for agreement or refusal to do what you ask. Don't assume that they have agreed because you have forgotten they have a choice too. They may refuse your request.

Use **the stuck record technique**: this involves repeating a brief statement about what you want over and over.

If you don't want to do something, **just say 'no.'** Don't give lots of reasons.

Above all, **believe in yourself** and your ability to achieve, even when others shake their heads. Find out what you have to learn and meet the challenge if it's something you really want to do.

6. Life after work.

Retirement is not only about **new opportunities** and having a **life after work** but also coming to terms, positively, with getting older and dealing with illness and infirmity, which may go along with the aging process.

Having a positive mind-set is important at this stage in life, but don't deny that getting older may have a negative effect on you. However, there are opportunities for new experiences and something positive to learn, even from a negative event.

If you are someone well-known in your working role, this is the time to discover who you are beneath the professional facade as you move away from those roles and identity.

As you **explore a life after work**, you need to believe that it is not only possible but also can be amazing. Instead of procrastinating with excuses about being upset because you don't want to leave work, be confident that things will turn out fine for you.

Whatever you want to do, **stop making excuses** that you can't do what you want to do because you: are too old, too fat, not clever enough, don't know how, don't have time, not that sort of person, or wouldn't be able to make a difference.

Decide this is the time in your life when you won't delay any more and you will do whatever you need to do to make your dreams come true.

Are you willing to **take a leap of faith** and change habits of a lifetime in order to have the life you dream of? If so, what do you have to change?

To **achieve your dreams and live the life you want**, you have to:

- Change the way you think about yourself.
- Change what you believe about yourself.
- Do what your inner self wants to do

As you approach retirement, with feelings of apprehension, excitement about what your next phase of life will bring, and wondering what it might mean for you, you have the chance to choose to live a different sort of life. You might be energised thinking about this possibility, or you may be dreading the changes when your work routine no longer dominates your life.

When you retire, the biggest problem you may meet with is that there is **too much choice** about what you can do. At first you may become bored when you haven't got enough to do because you no longer have the daily routine of work done for many years and you believe that it will be difficult to fill your day with useful activities.

However, the truth is that there are a huge number of things to do when you no longer must go to work. The biggest problem for you is deciding which of those things you are going to do. You could end up either hardly doing anything or doing far too much and becoming exhausted.

Here is what you can do to help you solve this problem:

Write what you really love doing: Ask yourself what you always wanted to learn about. You can research whether there are courses to enroll in so you can spend some valuable time improving your skills.

Decide what physical activities you like taking part in: This is a good time to swim regularly, attend exercise classes, practice Yoga or T'ai chi, or ride your bicycle every day. From the list you've made, pick two or three and explore these. Decide which day or days you will do those, whether you can do them on your own or if you need to find a companion or a class, and plan your week.

Find a balance between doing nothing and doing too much: Remember that your energy levels may not be as high as they were years ago, but don't let your biological age put you off the activity which you want to do.

See the funny side of life: Avoid getting stressed by things which you can't influence, have fun, try new things, make friends and be sure that you laugh every day. There is no advantage in getting overstressed because your retirement is a time to enjoy life, learn new skills and reflect on all the things that have brought you to where you find yourself now.

7. Plans into action.

If you use the excuse of age for not taking on the challenge of doing what you really want to do, then think again. If you think you are too old to change, then reflect on this: your joints may be stiff, but it's the inflexibility of your mind rather than your body that stops you from changing your life. When you retire from work, you have the ideal opportunity to do the things you always said you were too busy to do.

Become more aware about what might stop you now that you have more time. It's common to be scared about what others say or how they react when you do things differently. That's why it's so important to talk to as many people who might be affected by your changes and explain what you plan. It may surprise you at how they support and encourage you, and your fears may be ungrounded.

Spend a few hours listening to what you and others say in day-to-day conversation. Notice the words used, and the assumptions made. Do you hear yourself saying 'I'm no good at so and so,' or 'I'm dreading tomorrow,' or 'It's an awful journey to get from A to B' or 'I can't do that, what will they think of me!' Be aware of what you say and change your language to be more positive. Rather than 'I don't want'...say 'I want'...

Compose **affirmations** in relation to your goals. Affirmations are positive statements in the present tense starting with 'I am...' The statement should be as if what you want has already happened.

Write a paragraph about your life as if you wake up and your life has become the way you want it. Say where you are, what you see and hear, how you feel and who is with you. Read this every day and notice how your life changes to what you describe.

You really can change your life.

You've been telling people for years about **all the things you plan to do** when you retire, when you have more time. If you've been thinking about change for some time but not actually doing anything, then the first strategy for preparing yourself for action is recognising you can do whatever you set your mind to (well, almost anything).

However, it's also a time to come to terms with the way you may sabotage yourself by assumptions about your own abilities and how others will react to you.

You need to separate beliefs from reality. How can you do this? Start by asking:

- what evidence have I for this assumption?
- how do I know how someone will react?
- how do I know what life will be like?

It's very common to make assumptions about other people and the way they react to a situation, when it is an assumption, without evidence.

Assumptions are a way not to do something.

When you enter this **new phase of your life**, of a life after work, the first step is to prepare yourself:

- What do you have to do in order to start smoothly and continue onwards and upwards?
- How will you handle difficult situations without the routines of work?
- Do you worry about finding enough to do?
- Have you forgotten about your own health and well-being?
- Would you like to enjoy a life after work?
- Are you looking forward to having enough time to enjoy your friends and family?
- Would you like to spend quality time with your partner, or do you wonder what it will be like to be in each other's company for so much more of the time?
- Do you hope you will have the energy, motivation and enthusiasm for things you used to love to do but have been too busy or too exhausted to do?

8. Ways to stay busy.

Help other people: Volunteering in whatever way you feel able is a great way to spend time when you retire. Volunteer to work for a conservation project, show people around a stately home or befriend people who are lonely.

Help your family: If you have grandchildren, there will be plenty of opportunities to be involved with them, especially if they live nearby. You could babysit and give their parents a chance to have a few hours to go out for the evening and use the opportunity to get to know your grandchildren.

Learn a language: If you plan to travel, it's flattering to the locals if you can say a few words in their language.

Join a gym: Keeping your body active is important after you retire and this is a way to ensure you strengthen your muscles and joints. You might prefer to dance or join an exercise to music class or yoga to have a similar outcome.

Join a walking club: This is a great way to combine increasing your fitness by regular hiking and also having a sociable time meeting other people who also enjoy walking.

Join a choir, or music group: If you enjoy singing or playing an instrument or want to learn either of these skills, retirement is the time to indulge yourself.

Do something creative: Find workshops, courses or books and discover creativity, in activities such as painting drawing, photography or craft making, whichever you feel drawn to.

Getting engrossed in something creative is a way to let go of any day-to-day worries and become absorbed in what you are doing.

Read books: Make a resolution to read regularly whether this is to keep up to date with the news or to get to grips with piles of unread books you may have accumulated or have on a wish list to read someday.

Clear your clutter: Take it room by room or even cupboard-by-cupboard and clear away what you no longer need or want. Throw it away, give it to charity or sell it and get more space in your life.

Go on holiday: See fresh places, learn new customs and open your mind to another part of the world.

Enjoy yourself: When the day comes and you no longer must go to work, life may seem a little strange at first because there is no more routine of getting up and going to work each day, nor does someone else dictate the way you must spend the bulk of your days. Instead, enjoy your new life!

9. Finding your purpose.

Being aware of your purpose helps you decide what to do during your retirement so you don't fritter away your days. There are things which need to be done day by day such as shopping, cooking and other routine domestic tasks and there is the bigger purpose of your life: the reason you are here, and it's helpful to find out what it is so that you can work towards it as you go about your tasks every day.

How can you discover your purpose? Take some paper and write at the bottom of it three things you love to do, or three things that make you feel fantastic.

Starting with the first one, ask yourself 'When I .... (whatever you started with) ... what does that do for me?

You reply: 'it makes me ... ' and write above the first phrase what you said. Continue asking yourself the question and making an upward ladder of what each thing you say does for you. Eventually, you come to a stop or may loop back to something you said already.

Then (and it may not be until you have about 10 things written), go to the next thing that you love to do and repeat the process. Then so it again with number three.

You will then have a paper filled with the essence of the reasons that you enjoy doing certain things. Look for similarities between the lists and notice any sense in your body when you read through the top words. When you feel the emotion, the excitement, as you read the words, then you have found your purpose.

Ask yourself, 'In order to achieve my purpose, which is... what do I need to do?' How will I do it? Where, when and how? You already have discovered the 'Why?'

Then everything else in your life becomes aligned and you understand your motivation for doing what you do and why some things seem to flow while others that are not your purpose seem to be tiresome and irritating.

When you consider doing something new ask yourself if it fits in with your purpose in life because as you get older it feels good to do things which are so aligned and you don't need to be doing too much which is uncomfortable or lacking in that purpose.

Connect your purpose to your sense of self and self-esteem. Manage change in your life so much better when you are clear about your life's purpose. This is a step further than goal setting, which some people find quite difficult to do because they don't feel motivated to achieve the goal they set themselves.

However, once you are clear about your life purpose, the goals became clearer because they are the way you can achieve: they are the steps you need to take to move towards your purpose. Finding your life purpose is important at whatever stage of life you are. By identifying your purpose, you will gain clarity about what you are doing and why.

Exploring to find your life's purpose can be very exciting and rewarding and you will know why certain things are so important to you. You will gain clarity about what you need to do to achieve and how to spend your time. Your life will take on more meaning.

10. Get sorted.

Some people love being retired, yet others get extremely fed up. They miss the comradeship of work and the routine they had.

Here are some ways you can become more fed up and frustrated when you retire.

Don't plan what to do when you retire. Maybe you believe you will automatically know how to spend your day when you retire. However, after a lifetime of work, you may find it's difficult to decide what to do each day. Before you know it, days, weeks, months and finally years pass and you waste a lot of time. It's not too late to make plans about what you'll do during your retirement. You could follow where your spirit leads you, but may find that unless you make plans, it is more likely that you will become more and more fed up.

Only have friends connected to your work. You find that all your friends are people who worked with you. That means your friendship with those people relates to sharing what goes on at work. When you leave you find, with time, you have less and less in common and this is a formula for becoming more and more frustrated and bored.

Don't make new friends: Reverse this and make the effort to meet others by joining clubs, going to adult education classes and meeting new people not connected with your working life.

Never take time to learn anything different: You can guarantee that you will become more and more fed-up during retirement if you have never learnt anything about life except for things you had to learn in relation to your work. Find out what classes there are and start to open your mind to new opportunities.

Don't have any hobbies: By spending all your time at work you will have perfected the art of not doing anything else except working, watching television, eating and sleeping. This is the perfect formula for being very fed up when you are retired. Remember what you used to enjoy and promise yourself that you will find others so you make new friends as well as keeping your mind and body active.

There are many ways to get yourself and your life more organised. This is important when you retire. Life after work brings you new opportunities so if you are wasting time regularly find how to use your day more efficiently and effectively to fulfil some or all of your long-held ambitions and also explore new possibilities.

Plan your day the previous evening. This is one way to get more order into your life. However, if you don't like an imposed schedule, which may bring back memories of working with tight demands on your time, you may prefer to greet each day anew with a little idea at the start of it where it and your spirit will lead you.

However, it's worth trying and noticing how much more you can achieve each day. It can be a great motivator when you spend a few moments each evening thinking about and then deciding about what you want to get done the following day.

Be realistic: You know what you are capable of doing so set yourself tasks which you know you can easily complete in the time you have available. It's important to be practical about this.

Be specific: Avoid being vague about what you want to do. Rather than deciding something like 'continue with clearing clutter,' try instead to specify precisely what you will get done.

Write it down: The other important thing to remember is to make a note about whatever you decide to do. The mere act of writing something merges it in your mind, and you will be more likely to do it.

Strike a balance: Be aware of aiming too high or aiming too low when deciding what you want to get done the following day. When you aim too low, you can always do more and so feel very pleased with yourself, whereas aiming too high can lead you to feel frustrated and as if you have failed.

Designate specific times for yourself: You may have had years of too little exercise and eating unhealthy food during your working life. Don't let your increased leisure time lead you to eating more and exercising less. Take the opportunities you have to increase your health and well-being.

If you are feeling bored with not having a routine, here are some ways that you can prevent boredom, a fear that people have before they've actually retired. However, being bored after you finish work is a real possibility, especially if you find it difficult to **let go of your working identity.** It is important to understand that **'life after work' is a new stage of your life.** There may be a **period for transition** from your life from someone who goes out to work every day to your life as a retired person.

Inevitably, you will **develop a new identity** in your life after work. Yes, part of you is the same as it was before, but a large part of you changes and this is something you may need to work at. Since retirement is an opportunity to **explore new ways of living** your life, then it is also a chance to face the way you view what's happening around you.

Things that used to be overwhelmingly important take on a lesser significance after you've retired. You may wonder why you put up with so many things during your working life and understand how important other aspects of life are. These may be to do with your family and friends, becoming **more involved in community activities**, and also **doing things for yourself**, whether pursuing hobbies long since forgotten, or being more aware about how important it is to **look after your own health and well-being.**

To stop being bored when you retire you must **take an active role** and **decide what it is you really would like to do** now that you no longer have work commitments, because until you decide what it is you want then it will be more difficult to achieve it. Once you've decided what you'd like to spend your time doing **then make the necessary plans** to actually do it.

Find out about local facilities and classes in your area that are related to the things you'd like to do. Sometimes you can't just jump from your working persona into a new identity without learning something new. Learning at this time of your life is very exciting. It keeps your brain active and ensures that you will not be bored during your life after work.

11. Myths about retirement.

When you retire, you might have made some assumptions about life after work. Here are some of them.

1. You'll be bored without the routine of work: That depends, to some extent, on whether, during your working years, you developed interests apart from work. If so, you will have plenty to keep busy. There are classes to attend, clubs to join, and people who share your interests.

If you liked work so much and didn't develop other interests, then there will be opportunities, if you look for them, to be a mentor to others. To do the same work, but on an 'as and when' basis, perhaps filling in when someone is on holiday or unwell. This gives you the chance to cut down your commitments gradually and not have the strict obligation of having to work every day.

2. You cannot stay healthy: You may assume that you would become a 'couch potato' when you left work - someone who sits around all day watching television, eating and never exercising. Of course, if this is what you actually end up doing, then you will find your health deteriorates. However, in your life after work you are likely to have many years ahead of you in excellent health. You can help this by eating healthy meals, taking regular exercise such as walking for about thirty minutes each day, stopping smoking and limiting the amount of alcohol you drink.

3. You can't learn anything new. Change your mind-set to the benefits of lifelong learning and decide to learn something you knew nothing about or re-visit what you were interested in many years before. Most people, when they retire, keep their brain active and exercised by doing just that. Don't let your age put you off learning. Lifelong learning is important for keeping your mind and body active.

4. You'll have time to do plenty: You may find that once you leave work that some things you can fit into a day take longer to complete and you don't get as much done as you planned. Remember, although you have plenty of time, it's limited.

5. You will be fed up. Some people love being retired, yet others get extremely unhappy after some time because they miss the comradeship of work and the routine they had. Keep in touch with friends and family and also to make new friends. Social interaction is important to help with healthy aging.

6. You can't plan what to do when you retire. Maybe you believe you will know how to spend your day when you retire. However, after a lifetime of work routine, you may find it's difficult to decide what to do each day. Before you know it, days, weeks, months and finally years pass and you've wasted a lot of time.

7. Your life is over, so no point in doing anything new. However, it's not too late to make plans about what you'll do during your life after work.

8. Someone else will tell you what to do. You change your life in whatever way you want. Don't rely on others' ideas on how to spend your days.

9. Only have workplace friends. You may find that all your friends are people who worked with you. That means the friendship relates to sharing what goes on at work. When you leave you find that, with time, you have less and less in common and this is a formula for becoming more and more frustrated and bored. Instead, you could join clubs, go to adult education classes and meet new people.

10. There is no point in learning anything new. You can guarantee that you will become more and more fed-up during retirement if you have learnt nothing about life except for things in relation to your work. Open your mind to new opportunities and a different world opens up for you.

11. Don't have any hobbies. By spending all your time at work, you have perfected the art of not doing anything except working, watching television, eating and sleeping. This is the perfect formula for being fed up once you retire. Now is the perfect time to open yourself to new experiences. Remember what you used to enjoy and promise yourself that you will find others so you make new friends and keeping your mind and body active.

12. Retirement is the end of your working life.

You can continue to work, either in your current job or in a new one. There are many benefits to working in retirement, including the ability to stay active, to earn additional income, and to enjoy a sense of purpose.

13. You won't contribute to society in retirement.

You can still be active and contribute to society in retirement. There are many ways to do this, such as volunteering, working part-time, or starting a new business. This can help you stay mentally and physically active, and can also give you a sense of purpose. Retirement can be a great time to focus on your hobbies and interests, and there are plenty of ways to stay socially active as well.

14. Retirement means a life of leisure.

Retirement doesn't have to mean a life of leisure. It can be a time to pursue new interests and explore new hobbies. It can be a time to volunteer and give back to the community. It can be a time to travel and see fresh places. It can be a time to spend more time with family and friends. There are many ways to enjoy retirement, and it doesn't have to be all about relaxing.

15. You can't have a sense of purpose in retirement. Just because you're retired doesn't mean you can't have a sense of purpose. There are plenty of things you can do to stay active. You can volunteer, take up a new hobby, or even start your own business. Whatever you do, make sure you're doing something that brings you satisfaction. Retirement is a time to enjoy your life and do what you want to do. So, find something that brings you joy and stick with it. You'll be glad you did.

16. You can't be social in retirement. There are many ways to stay connected with friends and loved ones. You can volunteer, take classes, join social clubs, and take part in activities that interest you. You can also use technology to stay in touch, such as Zoom social media, and email.

17. You can't be active in retirement. Retirement doesn't have to mean sitting around the house all day. There are plenty of ways to stay engaged even after you retire.

12. Opportunities in life after work

Retirement gives you the chance to revisit neglected hobbies. You may have skills not used for years, because while working you didn't have the time to keep in touch or practice. You can get back to those things when you retire and learn anything to keep up to date with your chosen hobby or interest.

This is the time to **finish projects** you started years ago, get your clutter sorted and do what you didn't get around to before.

Retire and travel. If you always wanted to **travel and see the world** but never had the time available, make your plans and achieve them now.

Retirement is a time for you to stop whatever frustrates, annoys or upsets you. When you were working, you probably had to do things you didn't want to do, but in retirement you have choices: either let it go, or get someone else to do it.

Retirement is an opportunity to try new things. Try something creative or learn a new skill. There are plenty of courses available.

Retire and learn, because it's important that your brain remains active. You could learn a language or a musical instrument, take an Open University degree, or start a new hobby.

Retire and improve your fitness by regular exercise and using your car less. You have the advantage of a senior rail card and a bus pass if you live in the UK, so use these and enjoy visiting fresh places instead of driving. Walk more and your health benefits.

Retire and be more aware of the communities of which you are a part because when you have lots of interests, these will motivate you to be part of, and take an active role in your community.

Retire and join whatever appeals to you because that enables you to get involved and contribute. You are at a stage in your life when you have a lot to offer and it is satisfying to help others.

Retire and plan, because this avoids waking up and wondering what to do all day. Keep note of events you are interested in, films or plays you want to see. When you decide how to spend your time, you will be excited to get on with your plans.

Retire and keep in touch with family because whether they live nearby or on the other side of the world, it's important to communicate regularly.

Retire and meet old friends and make new ones because then you won't stay at home feeling sorry for yourself. Being retired is a great time to connect with people, especially if many of your friends are still working. Meeting people for a walk, a cup of tea or sharing a meal together helps to keep you healthy.

Retire and go to the beach to laze about, sunbathe, swim, read a good book and relax because you benefit from some exercise, the sea air and relaxation.

Retire and take part in a challenge to stretch yourself and train to get fit enough to climb a mountain, walk on glaciers or swim across the river because it's empowering to succeed in something challenging. There are challenges for many activities and places. Pick one you fancy and go for it. You'll feel great when you train for it and succeed and raise money for charity at the same time.

Retire and rest and relax with whatever you plan to do during your years after work, because it's important, you have time to be active and time to 'switch off' and just 'be'. Avoid the tendency amongst some people when they retire to continue the pace of their working day and feel guilty if they are not busy all the time.

Retire and be more active:

- **Join a club or group.** Whether it's a book club, a gardening club, or a group that meets to discuss current events, being a part of a club can help you.
- **Take up a new hobby.** Now is the perfect time to try something new. Whether it's painting, hiking, or bird watching, exploring a new hobby can help you stay active both mentally and physically.
- **Get involved in your community.** There are many ways to get involved in your community, such as volunteering, joining a local organisation, or running for office. Getting involved enables you to find the subjects that matter to you.
- **Travel.** Retirement is the perfect time to travel. Whether you take a long trip or visit a new city or country, traveling can help you see the world in a new way and can be a great way to stay active and engaged.
- **Stay connected with friends and family.** This is important at any age. Retirement is a great time to reconnect with old friends or to spend more time with

your family.

13. Make life easier.

When you look around at people who have retired, you may notice that there are those who find it extremely difficult to know what to do with themselves when they no longer have to go to work each day, and those who are excited and happy to do many new things in their lives.

What motivates this second group to get involved in new experiences?

They set goals: When you know what you want, then you know what you are working towards, and this is a powerful motivator. Do you remember how, when you were at work, you achieved much more when you had specific deadlines? Remember this in your life after work, be clear about what you want, and by when you want to achieve it.

They do something each day towards achieving: Instead of aiming to do everything all at once, decide on small steps you can do each day and by so doing, move towards what you want to achieve.

They keep their vision in mind. Even while only taking small steps, keep your vision in mind and keep telling yourself that these steps are bringing you nearer to it. Be even more strongly motivated if by involving other people and regularly discussing what you are aiming to achieve.

They look after themselves: Be aware of how important it is to look after yourself when you retire by eating healthily, exercising regularly, learning new things and being open to new experiences. In this way, you will remain able to move forward towards achieving your goals because you will have enough energy to achieve everything you set out to do.

They celebrate their progress with positive feedback: As you move towards achieving what you want, acknowledge your positive progress and celebrate this. Avoid negative self-talk because this will hinder your progress. Not only celebrate progress with positive affirmations, but also encourage others to give you constructive feedback.

They manage their time. It can be a challenge when you retire to manage time effectively. Time management may have been a constant source of stress when you were working, and it can still be an issue when you no longer have to go to work. The challenge in retirement is using your time effectively and taking advantage of the new opportunities available to you.

They get rid of irritating tasks: You have been saying to yourself for years that when you retire, you would get lots of minor jobs done. So, either spend a few days doing just that or designate a set time each day until they are done and dusted. Don't let them take over all your time: there are so many new things you could do now instead.

They plan: If you flit from one task to another throughout the day, then you will benefit from doing things more efficiently. Do similar tasks together so you don't have to repeat journeys whether these are inside or outside.

They get rid of clutter: When you retire, you are entering a new stage in your life, a time to re-assess and re-group and think back over your life and forward to the rest of it. It's a great time to sort out what you want to keep and clear out unwanted and unnecessary clutter. You find that clearing physical space will also clear emotional clutter, too.

They choose how to spend the day: Without the routine of work, you have the chance to make more choices, especially in the way you want to spend each day, and may include more involvement with friends and family, perhaps looking after and enjoying the company of grandchildren. Be clear about your boundaries, however, and about how much you will do.

They choose with whom to spend time: You have a choice too about with whom to spend time. It's easy to get into an ongoing habit of, for example, friends who visit you, then they invite you back and so on ad infinitum. If you enjoy their company, then that's fine. If you dread seeing them and don't enjoy their company, then just say 'no' and stop. Choose to spend time with friends and family for their good company. Don't forget it's also important to spend some time with yourself, doing whatever you enjoy.

They are open to new opportunities: Without work routines when you retire; you have days stretching ahead of you and opportunities to do many things you've been dreaming about for years.

Do you resolve to follow some, or all the habits listed and look forward to a great life after work?

14. The advantages of retiring.

Life after work is a new phase of your life. You will find doors opening offering new opportunities and it can boost the way you experience the joys of life if you retire. The trouble is, many people are scared at the idea of not working because they think there won't be anything to do, when they retire.

Here are some of the advantages of retiring from your current work:

The opportunity to start a completely different career or business: There is nothing to stop you from doing what you wish you'd done years ago. Many people decide to apply for jobs in a completely different industry, or start their own business, possibly working from home.

Being able to do whatever you always dreamt of doing: You may have been saying to people "if only I had the time...". When you retire, you have the time to do those things you always talked about.

Becoming more involved with your community: You will have the time and the opportunity to be involved in what's going on in your community. If you have a residents' association, take a more active part in that or join other committees so that people in your community can benefit from your experience.

Join community activities. Become aware of the communities of which you are a part, because this will motivate you to be part of and take an active role.

Meet members of your family more frequently, renew old friendships and make new friends: If you've had a busy working life then you may have neglected family visits, and keeping in touch with friends so when you retire keep in touch more frequently.

Be more creative: You can paint, draw, photograph, sing or play music. Do whatever you feel drawn to do and don't restrict yourself by other people's rules in relation to your creativity. Enjoy the process.

Get your life sorted: After a lifetime of being busy, you now get rid of what you no longer need. Clear cupboards, donate to charities and throw things away.

Travel: There are wonderful opportunities to visit wherever you want to go.

Think about your life. When you retire, the biggest problem you may encounter is that there is too much choice about what you can do. At first you may be bored because you think you haven't got enough to do when you no longer have the routine of work. You may believe that it will be difficult to fill your day with useful activities.

However, there are a huge number of things you can do when you no longer must go to work, so the biggest problem for you may be to decide which of those things you are going to do. Some people have such a challenge with that decision that they end up hardly starting anything or undertaking far too much and becoming exhausted.

Review how your life is changing. If you are setting unachievable or unrealistic goals which you are expecting to achieve with very little effort, then reap the benefits of thinking over the way you'd like life to be in retirement.

How can you live with the challenges of life as a retired person? If you spent a large part of your day in front of a computer and your leisure time watching television, then your fitness may be inadequate. Perhaps you know this very well and from time to time joined a gym or played a sport but got fed up or too tired to continue after a few weeks. Make the decision to do regular exercise so that you remain fit enough to enjoy your life after work for many years.

What will you do to enjoy your life after work?

It's a time to reassess your life and decide how you want to spend the rest of it. Some people think of it as a prolonged holiday and become extremely lazy and do nothing very much.

If you have left a busy job, you may find that when you eventually retire, you feel exhausted and find it difficult to find the motivation to do anything except sit around, eat and watch television all day.

Although it's fine to take a bit more relaxation time when you retire, you are fitter and healthier if you get on with your life and develop new interests, make new friends and go to places that you have never been to before. Make a list of all those things you wish you had time for when you were still working.

After many years of doing something similar every day, your self-esteem may be at rock bottom and you may think that you can only do things related to your work experience. However, when people retire and develop the confidence and courage to try something entirely new, or something they always wished they knew how to do, are surprised to find they have many talents. Doing something entirely new is very energising and opens your mind to possibilities.

What you decide to do after you let go of the work routine is, to a large extent, up to you. It may be related to a long-forgotten hobby which you wish to take up again or other interests which you had no time to take part in when you were busy at work.

As you get older, your health and well-being become more important and this is the time to look at your lifestyle in relation to your state of health and wellness, deciding what you must do now to increase your chances of a healthy old age.

As always, it is about balance between what you do for yourself and what you do because of pressure from others.

If you can match both demands on your time and energy, so much the better for you. However, if not, be aware of your own internal reactions to doing those things you love to do against doing something because of an obligation. If the latter leaves you feeling drained or stressed, then it is important to confront this and make adjustments so that whatever you do gives you a feeling of excitement and anticipation.

Think about your beliefs and values: your core beliefs. Yours may have come from parents and teachers. Are they still valid or do you need to discard some, like the tooth fairy? Beliefs from long ago can influence your actions today. If there is something you want to do but find it difficult to take the vital first step, ask yourself what's stopping you, what's the worst thing that could happen if you did that? Discarding old beliefs and taking on new ones is the vital first step you need to take to get your life on a fresh track.

Increase your skills and competencies: Do you need to learn something? What do you already know? Have you any transferable skills?

These may be in relation not only to your working life and professional skills, but also those you have in your domestic and social life.

What would be useful when you move into the life you really want?

When and how will you go about acquiring the new skills which you may need?

Can you ever know it all?

Don't wait until you are 'perfect'. Start as soon as possible. Learn as you go along and adapt to the new circumstances.

Lifelong learning is important to keep your brain active and to enable you to let your life experiences and learning mature. You are never too old to learn something new!

Life is like a spreadsheet, so change one thing and everything else changes. Have you ever used a spreadsheet to work out the effect of, for example, paying different amounts of money each month? By altering the amount saved, or the amount of interest earned each month, you notice how all the totals change too.

There is an interconnection between the parts of any system. Changing something in one part of your life will influence other areas of your life, even if apparently unconnected. If you don't know what to do, then tidying some cupboards and throwing away some things you no longer need seem to create some space for new things to come into your life.

15. Personal experience

It took me over a year to decide to leave Medicine, the profession I'd been part of for over thirty years. Part of my hesitation to take the action I knew I wanted was because of my fears about retirement. I worried about the loss of my identity and of a lack of routine in my life. I wondered how I would spend my days without the imposed routine of regular employment. It was only after I retired, I realised that life after work is exciting.

I was overjoyed to find my fears were ungrounded. There were so many opportunities for learning new skills, for developing others, and for exploring the world.

Both by the opportunities available on entering the 'third age' and some amazing people have inspired me. They don't regard retirement as 'the end of the road' but a time for new and exciting opportunities.

I hope to inspire and motivate you to enjoy your life after work, too. When you reach the time to retire, it's important to look at your life as if from the outside and re-assess where you want it to take you from now onwards. Your life involves others, not just you, so whatever you wish to do may also affect them, your partner, your friends, family, your community, and you.

Finally

Thank-you so much for supporting my work by reading this book.

If you enjoyed it, please let me know by leaving a brief review on the website from which you bought it

It only takes about 30 seconds and is incredibly useful for me as an independent author, and it helps other readers find my books.

Thanks for taking the time to do this. I really, really appreciate it.

Don't miss out!

Visit the website below and you can sign up to receive emails whenever Susan Kersley publishes a new book. There's no charge and no obligation.

https://books2read.com/r/B-A-EFNC-QOJLB

BOOKS 2 READ

Connecting independent readers to independent writers.

Did you love *Life After Work*? Then you should read *Get Ready for Retirement*[1] by Susan Kersley!

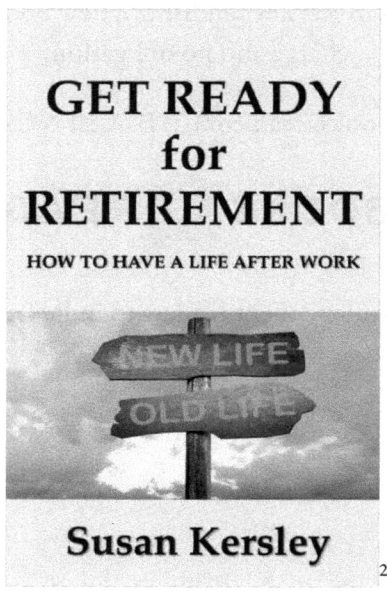
[2]

Are you apprehensive about having a life after work? Do you wonder how you'll manage without the routine of work? This book will enable you to get ready forretirement.

This book provides you with simple strategies in an easy-to-read format and a step-by-step approach so you can enjoy life after work and make the changes you want to make.

Susan Kersley is a retired Medical Practitioner who became a Life Coach and Writer.

---

1. https://books2read.com/u/bPEXl3

2. https://books2read.com/u/bPEXl3

She is the author of personal development books for doctors including 'Prescription for Change for doctors who want a life,' 'ABC of Change for Doctors,' and 'Life After Medicine.She has also published novels: 'Pills and Pillboxes' and 'Connection Deception.'

Read more at https://susankersley.co.uk.

Also by Susan Kersley

A Novel
Pills and Pillboxes
Connection Deception

Books about Weight Management
Change Your Mind, Change Your Weight
Weight Loss Success
Mind Over Weight

Books for Doctors
ABC of Change for Doctors
Life After Medicine
Prescription for Change
Lifestyle Coaching for Doctors
The Busy Doctor's Guide: Improve your Work-Life Balance
Work-Life Balance for Doctors
Simple Ways to Meet the Challenges of Working as a Doctor
Meet the Challenges of Working as a Doctor

Retirement Books
Get Ready for Retirement
Retirement: Back to Basics
Life After Work

Self-help Books
How to Have a Balanced Life
69 Easy Ways to Change Your life
Connect and Change
Coping With New Year Resolutions
How to Change Your Life
Improve Your Work Life Balance
More Time for You Now
15 Ways to Change Your Life
16 Ways to Change Your Life
Epiphany for Change

Watch for more at https://susankersley.co.uk.

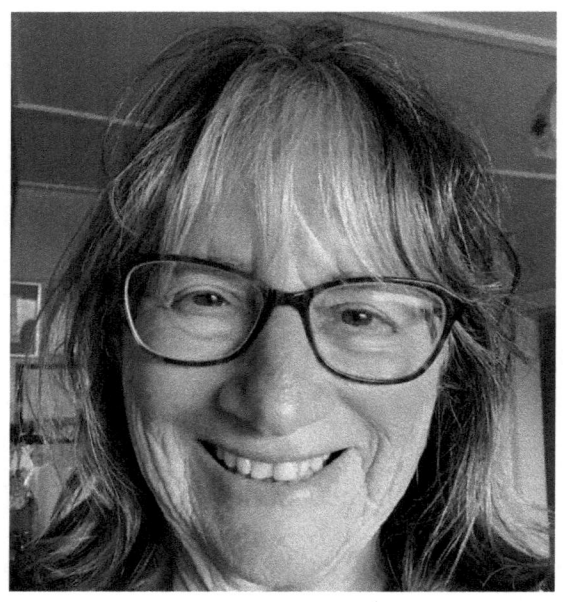

About the Author

Susan Kersley has written personal development and self-help books for doctors and others, and books about retirement and novels.

She was a doctor for thirty years and then left Medicine to be a Life Coach..

Now retired, she is updating her books and writing more. Please visit her website https://susankersley.co.uk

If you enjoyed this book, **please take a moment to leave a review.** Reviews are so important for independent authors.

Read more at https://susankersley.co.uk.

www.ingramcontent.com/pod-product-compliance
Ingram Content Group UK Ltd.
Pitfield, Milton Keynes, MK11 3LW, UK
UKHW020647071025
8268UKWH00040B/579